AI Mental Health & Emotional Regulation

How Artificial Intelligence Stabilizes Mood, Trauma & Anxiety

By Joe Correa

Published by Live Stronger Faster

This book is for educational and informational purposes only. The author and publisher are not engaged in rendering legal, financial, or other professional advice. Readers should consult a qualified professional before making any financial decisions.

First Edition

Table of Contents

Introduction

Mental health has long been treated as something fragile, mysterious, and painfully slow to repair. For generations, anxiety, depression, trauma, and emotional dysregulation were approached as conditions to be managed rather than systems to be retrained. People were told to cope, suppress, or endure, often without understanding what was actually happening inside their nervous system and brain. This book begins with a different premise entirely: that emotional stability is not a fixed trait, but a dynamic neurological process, and that artificial intelligence is now providing tools powerful enough to help the brain relearn safety, balance, and regulation at unprecedented speed.

At its core, emotional regulation is a neurological skill. It is shaped by neural pathways, reinforced by repetition, and influenced by how the brain interprets threat, memory, and prediction. Trauma, anxiety, and mood disorders are not merely emotional experiences; they are patterns embedded in the brain's circuitry. When the nervous system remains stuck in survival mode, even long after danger has passed, the mind reacts as if the past is still happening. Artificial intelligence offers a new way to interrupt this loop, not by forcing change, but by adapting to the brain's signals and gently guiding it toward healthier states.

Unlike traditional mental health interventions that rely heavily on retrospective discussion or static treatment models, AI operates in real time. It observes patterns, responds dynamically, and adjusts continuously. This matters deeply for emotional healing, because emotions do not arise in isolation. They are responses to perceived input, shaped by memory, expectation, and bodily sensation. AI systems are uniquely capable of tracking these variables simultaneously, identifying emotional triggers as they emerge, and helping retrain the brain's response before it spirals into overwhelm.

One of the most profound shifts explored in this book is the movement from reactive mental health care to proactive emotional training. Instead of waiting for anxiety attacks, depressive episodes, or emotional shutdowns to occur, AI-driven systems can identify early warning signals in speech patterns, typing rhythms, sleep data, heart rate variability, and behavioral changes. These systems do not diagnose in the traditional sense; they detect deviation from baseline and respond with personalized interventions that help stabilize emotional states before distress becomes debilitating.

Emotional regulation is deeply tied to prediction. The brain is constantly forecasting what will happen next, using past experiences to shape present reactions. Trauma disrupts this system, teaching the brain to expect danger even in safe environments. Anxiety amplifies uncertainty, while depression narrows prediction toward hopeless outcomes. Artificial intelligence excels at pattern recognition and prediction, making it uniquely suited to help recalibrate how the brain anticipates emotional outcomes. By providing consistent, adaptive feedback, AI can help retrain prediction pathways so the brain learns safety, flexibility, and emotional range again.

This book also explores how AI is transforming therapy from something that happens occasionally to something that supports the mind continuously. AI-driven mental health tools are not replacements for human connection; they are extensions of support that fill the gaps between sessions, moments, and crises. They provide grounding prompts, emotional labeling, cognitive reframing, and nervous system regulation exercises precisely when they are needed most. For many individuals, this continuity is the missing link that allows real progress to occur.

Another critical dimension addressed in these pages is personalization. Emotional healing is not one-size-fits-all. Two people can experience the same event and develop entirely different emotional patterns based on genetics, history, and nervous system sensitivity. AI thrives in personalization. It learns how a specific individual reacts to stress, which interventions are effective, and when support should be intensified or softened. Over time, this creates a feedback loop in which emotional regulation becomes easier, faster, and more intuitive.

The ethical responsibility of using AI in mental health is also central to this discussion. Emotional data is among the most sensitive forms of information a human can generate. This book addresses transparency, consent, privacy, and the importance of designing AI systems that empower rather than manipulate. The goal of AI-assisted emotional regulation is not control, but autonomy—the ability for individuals to understand their inner world and regain agency over their emotional responses.

As emotional intelligence becomes increasingly valuable in a fast-moving, high-stimulation world, the ability to regulate mood, stress, and trauma is no longer optional. Burnout, emotional exhaustion, and chronic anxiety are not signs of weakness; they are signals that the brain is overloaded and under-supported. Artificial intelligence, when applied thoughtfully, offers a scalable way to provide that support without stigma, delay, or overwhelm.

This book is written for anyone who has ever felt trapped by their emotions, confused by their reactions, or frustrated by slow progress. It is for clinicians, technologists, researchers, and everyday individuals who want to understand how the mind heals when given the right feedback. It does not promise instant fixes or emotional perfection. Instead, it offers a grounded, science-informed vision of how AI can help the brain do what it has always been capable of: learning, adapting, and returning to balance.

By the time you reach the end of this book, you will understand emotional regulation not as a personality trait, but as a trainable neurological process. You will see anxiety and trauma not as permanent scars, but as patterns that can be softened and reshaped. Most importantly, you will see artificial intelligence not as something cold or mechanical, but as a tool that—when designed with care—can help the human mind feel safer, steadier, and more whole in an increasingly complex world.

Chapter 1

The Emotional Brain as a Trainable System

The human emotional system was never designed for the pace, volume, and intensity of the modern world. Long before screens, notifications, constant information flow, and chronic uncertainty, the brain evolved to respond to immediate physical threats and short-term social dynamics. Emotions such as fear, anger, sadness, and joy were survival signals, designed to mobilize the body quickly and then subside once the situation resolved. What has changed is not the brain's hardware, but the environment it must now navigate, an environment that rarely allows the nervous system to fully return to baseline.

Emotional dysregulation occurs when the brain's threat-detection and emotional-response systems remain active longer than necessary. Anxiety persists when the amygdala continues to flag danger without resolution. Trauma embeds itself when emotional memory networks link past experiences to present stimuli. Depression emerges when prediction systems repeatedly forecast negative outcomes and suppress motivation. These are not character flaws or moral weaknesses. They are learned neural patterns reinforced through repetition, stress, and lack of corrective feedback. The key insight that underpins this entire book is that emotional regulation is not a static state but a dynamic, trainable process. Just as muscles adapt to repeated movement, emotional circuits strengthen or weaken based on how frequently they are activated and how they are resolved. When emotional responses are left unchecked, the brain learns that heightened states are normal. When emotional responses are gently interrupted, reframed, and resolved, the brain learns flexibility. Artificial intelligence enters this process not as an external controller, but as a responsive mirror that helps the brain observe and reshape its own patterns.

Traditional approaches to mental health have often relied on delayed reflection. A person experiences emotional distress, time passes, and later they attempt to analyze what happened. While insight is valuable, it often arrives too late to influence the original emotional cascade. AI systems operate differently. They engage during the moment emotional patterns are forming. By recognizing changes in language, behavior, tone, pace, and physiological signals, AI can detect emotional shifts before they escalate into full dysregulation.

The emotional brain operates largely below conscious awareness. Many reactions happen milliseconds before rational thought engages. This is why telling someone to "calm down" rarely works. The nervous system has already decided that vigilance is required. AI-assisted emotional regulation works by slowing this process down. It introduces micro-pauses, reframes interpretations, and offers grounding inputs that allow higher cortical regions to re-engage before emotional responses become overwhelming.

Another critical concept explored in this chapter is emotional labeling. Neuroscience research has shown that naming emotions accurately reduces amygdala activation and increases prefrontal regulation. However, many individuals struggle to identify what they are feeling in real time. AI systems trained on emotional language patterns can assist with this process, offering suggestions that help individuals recognize whether they are experiencing fear, grief, frustration, shame, or overstimulation. This clarity alone can significantly reduce emotional intensity.

Emotional regulation is also deeply connected to prediction and expectation. The brain is constantly estimating what will happen next based on past experiences. When someone has lived through repeated stress or trauma, the brain learns to expect negative outcomes even in neutral situations. AI can help retrain these predictive models by offering alternative interpretations, highlighting cognitive distortions, and reinforcing evidence-based reframes that gradually expand the brain's emotional range. Importantly, AI does not replace human therapy, connection, or introspection. Instead, it fills the spaces where support is often missing. It provides consistency, immediacy, and adaptability. It can respond at three in the morning when anxiety spikes, or during a stressful workday when emotional overload builds quietly. Over time, these small interventions compound, teaching the brain that regulation is possible and safety can be restored.

This chapter establishes the foundation for everything that follows. Emotional stability is not about eliminating difficult emotions. It is about restoring choice, flexibility, and resilience. Artificial intelligence offers a new category of tools that operate at the speed of emotion itself, helping the brain relearn balance not through force, but through guided adaptation. What comes next is not emotional perfection, but emotional literacy and control rooted in neuroscience, feedback, and intelligent support.

The Day the Noise Finally Quieted

Daniel had lived with anxiety for so long that he no longer remembered what calm felt like. It wasn't the dramatic kind that caused panic attacks or sent him to the emergency room. It was quieter, more constant, like a low electrical hum running through his chest from the moment he woke up until he finally fell asleep from exhaustion. He had learned to function with it, to work, to smile, to appear composed, even as his thoughts raced endlessly beneath the surface.

Every decision felt heavy. Every silence felt loaded. His brain scanned conversations for hidden meanings, replayed old mistakes without mercy, and projected futures that never seemed to end well. Therapy had helped him understand where some of it came from, but understanding hadn't stopped the sensations themselves. His body still reacted as if danger were always just around the corner.

What changed wasn't a breakthrough conversation or a sudden realization. It started with a small experiment, something his therapist suggested as an additional layer of support. An AI-based emotional regulation tool that responded to his journaling, messaging, and daily check-ins. Daniel was skeptical. He didn't want another app telling him how to feel. But he agreed to try it, promising himself he would quit if it felt invasive or artificial.

The first few days were uneventful. The system asked simple questions, reflected his language back to him, and occasionally suggested grounding exercises. What surprised him was the timing. The prompts appeared not when he was already overwhelmed, but just before. When his messages became shorter, more rigid, or more negative, the system responded with gentle curiosity. It asked what his body felt like. It offered words he hadn't considered. It slowed him down.

One afternoon, while sitting at his desk, Daniel felt the familiar tightness in his chest. His thoughts began spiraling toward an upcoming meeting he was convinced would go badly. Before the spiral fully took hold, a notification appeared. It mirrored his concern, named the emotion as anticipatory anxiety, and suggested a brief breathing pattern. He followed it, reluctantly at first, then with growing focus. The tightness softened. The thoughts didn't disappear, but they lost their urgency.

Over the next few weeks, something subtle shifted. Daniel began noticing his emotional patterns sooner. He recognized when his mind jumped ahead catastrophically. He learned to pause, label what was happening, and choose a response rather than being pulled along by habit. The AI didn't give him answers. It gave him space.

The most unexpected moment came one evening as he sat quietly on his couch, doing nothing in particular. For the first time in years, there was no buzzing in his chest, no mental noise demanding attention. Just silence. Not empty silence, but calm. Daniel realized then that his anxiety hadn't vanished. It had loosened its grip. His brain had learned, slowly and patiently, that it didn't need to stay on guard all the time. That night, as he reflected on the experience, Daniel understood something deeply important. Healing hadn't come from eliminating his emotions. It had come from learning to work with them in real time, with support that met him where he was. The noise didn't disappear forever, but it no longer controlled him. And for the first time in a long time, that felt like freedom.

Chapter 2

Trauma, Memory, and the Brain's Stuck Signals

Trauma is not defined by what happens to a person, but by what remains unresolved in the nervous system afterward. Two individuals can experience the same event, yet only one may carry its emotional imprint for years. This is because trauma is stored not as a narrative memory, but as a sensory and emotional pattern encoded deep within the brain. Sounds, images, sensations, and emotions become linked in ways that bypass conscious reasoning and reactivate the body as if the past were still present.

At the neurological level, trauma disrupts the brain's ability to distinguish between past and present. The amygdala becomes hypersensitive, scanning constantly for threat, while the hippocampus struggles to place memories in proper context. When these systems fall out of balance, the brain reacts reflexively. A tone of voice, a facial expression, or a moment of uncertainty can trigger the same physiological response that once accompanied real danger. The body reacts first, and the mind follows. Traditional trauma approaches often focus on revisiting memories, retelling stories, or attempting to cognitively reframe experiences. While these methods can be helpful, they do not always reach the level at which trauma is stored. The nervous system does not respond to logic alone. It responds to patterns, repetition, and safety signals delivered consistently over time. This is where artificial intelligence introduces a fundamentally new pathway for trauma recovery.

AI-assisted trauma regulation works by identifying when the nervous system is slipping into a trauma response before full activation occurs. Subtle changes in language, pacing, posture, breathing, and attention often precede conscious awareness of distress. AI systems trained on these signals can recognize early shifts and intervene gently, offering grounding cues that help the brain reorient to the present moment. This early intervention is critical because once the trauma response fully engages, it becomes much harder to interrupt.

Memory reconsolidation plays a central role in trauma healing. Each time a memory is recalled, it briefly becomes malleable before being stored again. If new emotional information is introduced during this window, the memory can be altered. AI systems can help facilitate this process by guiding individuals through recall experiences while maintaining emotional regulation, allowing traumatic memories to be updated with a sense of safety rather than fear. Another essential function of AI in trauma recovery is pacing. One of the greatest risks in trauma work is moving too fast. Overexposure can retraumatize, while avoidance can reinforce fear. AI systems can adapt dynamically, slowing down when stress indicators rise and offering distance when emotional intensity becomes too high. This responsiveness helps rebuild trust in the body's ability to process difficult material without becoming overwhelmed.

Trauma also fragments attention. Individuals often oscillate between hypervigilance and dissociation, either too alert or emotionally numb. AI-guided interventions help stabilize this swing by encouraging consistent engagement with present-moment awareness. Through repeated micro-interventions, the brain learns that it can remain grounded without needing to shut down or escalate.

Importantly, trauma recovery is not about erasing memory. It is about restoring choice. When the brain no longer reacts automatically, individuals regain the ability to respond intentionally. AI does not force resolution. It creates the conditions under which resolution becomes possible by reinforcing safety, predictability, and self-awareness.

This chapter establishes that trauma is not a life sentence written into the brain. It is a pattern that can be softened, reshaped, and integrated. Artificial intelligence, when designed with care and ethical responsibility, offers a steady companion in this process, one that supports healing not through pressure, but through intelligent presence and repetition.

When the Past Lost Its Grip

Maria avoided mirrors for years, not because she disliked her reflection, but because looking at herself made her feel exposed. She had learned long ago that safety came from staying small, unnoticed, and emotionally distant. The trauma she carried was not something she spoke about often. It lived instead in her body, in the way her shoulders tightened when someone stood too close, in the way her breath shortened during conflict, in the way her mind went blank whenever emotions ran high.

She had tried to explain it before, to therapists, to friends, even to herself. But words never quite captured what happened inside her. One moment she would be present, the next she would feel pulled somewhere else, detached from her surroundings, watching herself from a distance. It was as if her nervous system had learned a shortcut: disappear before things become too much.

When Maria began using an AI-supported trauma regulation tool, she did not expect much. She assumed it would feel mechanical, maybe even intrusive. Instead, it felt surprisingly quiet. The system did not ask her to explain her past. It simply observed how she interacted with it. It noticed when her responses became delayed, when her language flattened, when her attention drifted.

One evening, after a difficult conversation with a coworker, Maria felt herself slipping into that familiar numbness. Before she could fully disconnect, the system prompted her gently, asking her to notice where she felt tension in her body. She paused. For the first time, she stayed. She named the sensation. She breathed. The moment passed without pulling her under.

Over the following weeks, Maria began to experience something new. Her trauma responses still appeared, but they softened faster. She noticed the early signs before dissociation took hold. The AI did not tell her what to do. It reminded her that she had options. That she could slow down. That she could stay present without being overwhelmed.

The most powerful moment came unexpectedly. While recalling a memory she had long avoided, Maria felt fear rise, then something else alongside it: calm. The memory no longer hijacked her body. It felt distant, contained, no longer dangerous. She realized then that the past had not disappeared, but it had lost its authority.

Maria stood in front of a mirror that night and met her own eyes without flinching. For the first time, she felt anchored in the present. The trauma had shaped her, but it no longer defined her. And in that quiet recognition, she understood that healing was not about forgetting what happened. It was about teaching her nervous system that it was finally safe to move forward.

Chapter 3

Anxiety, Mood Cycles, and Real-Time Emotional Regulation

Anxiety is not the presence of fear, but the absence of certainty. It emerges when the brain's prediction systems fail to resolve ambiguity and instead default to vigilance. Unlike fear, which responds to immediate danger, anxiety lingers, scanning for threats that may never materialize. The emotional brain becomes trapped in a loop of anticipation, constantly preparing for outcomes that remain unresolved. Over time, this state becomes self-reinforcing, teaching the nervous system that alertness is safer than rest.

Mood instability often follows the same pattern. Emotional highs and lows are not random fluctuations, but reflections of how the brain interprets safety, control, and expectation. When prediction systems repeatedly anticipate negative outcomes, motivation declines and emotional range narrows. When anticipation spikes without resolution, anxiety dominates. The brain is not malfunctioning in these states; it is attempting to protect itself with the information it has learned.

Artificial intelligence introduces a powerful shift in how anxiety and mood cycles can be regulated because it operates within the same temporal window as emotional activation. Anxiety does not announce itself politely. It builds quietly, through small physiological changes, altered breathing, tightened muscles, accelerated thoughts, and subtle language shifts. AI systems trained on these signals can recognize emotional escalation long before it reaches conscious awareness, allowing intervention while regulation is still possible.

One of the most significant advantages of AI-assisted emotional regulation is immediacy. Traditional coping strategies often rely on recall, requiring individuals to remember techniques while already overwhelmed. AI systems respond in the moment, offering prompts, grounding cues, and reframes precisely when emotional patterns begin to shift. This timing trains the brain to associate regulation with activation, rather than after-the-fact correction.

Anxiety thrives on uncertainty, and AI excels at pattern clarification. By reflecting emotional data back to the user, AI helps externalize internal states. When emotions are observed rather than fused with identity, they lose intensity. The brain shifts from being inside the emotion to observing it. This change alone can significantly reduce anxiety by re-engaging the prefrontal cortex and restoring cognitive flexibility. Mood regulation also depends on rhythm. The nervous system responds to consistency and predictability. AI-driven tools provide stable, repeatable interventions that help smooth emotional cycles over time. Rather than dramatic emotional swings, the brain begins to settle into narrower, more manageable ranges. This does not eliminate emotion; it restores balance.

Another critical function of AI in anxiety regulation is reducing self-judgment. Many individuals experience secondary distress, anxiety about anxiety, or shame about emotional reactions. AI systems respond without judgment, creating a neutral space where emotions can be acknowledged without escalation. This absence of emotional friction allows regulation to occur more naturally and sustainably.

Importantly, AI does not attempt to eliminate anxious thoughts. It helps contextualize them. By identifying cognitive distortions, catastrophic projections, and repetitive loops, AI gently redirects attention toward present-moment data. Over time, this retrains the brain's predictive models, reducing the frequency and intensity of anxiety-driven responses.

This chapter establishes that anxiety and mood instability are not fixed traits or chemical accidents. They are learned responses shaped by experience, reinforcement, and interpretation. Artificial intelligence provides a responsive training environment in which the emotional brain can relearn safety, flexibility, and trust in real time. Regulation becomes not an emergency response, but a practiced skill embedded into daily life.

Learning to Trust the Quiet

Ethan had always been described as high-functioning. He met deadlines, maintained relationships, and appeared calm under pressure. What people didn't see was the constant tension beneath the surface, the endless mental rehearsals, the way his thoughts raced ahead of the present moment as if something terrible were always about to happen. His anxiety wasn't loud. It was relentless.

Every morning began with anticipation. What could go wrong today? What detail might he miss? What outcome might spiral beyond his control? His mind treated uncertainty as a threat, and rest as a risk. Even during moments of success, relief was brief. His brain quickly moved on to the next potential problem.

When Ethan began using an AI-based emotional regulation system, he did so reluctantly. He doubted that anything external could keep pace with his thoughts. But what surprised him was how little the system spoke, and how precisely it responded. It didn't interrupt his anxiety. It noticed it. During a work presentation one afternoon, Ethan felt the familiar tightening in his chest. His thoughts began racing toward worst-case scenarios. Before panic fully set in, a subtle prompt appeared, inviting him to slow his breathing and name what he was feeling. He complied almost automatically. The spiral paused. The moment passed.

Over the following weeks, Ethan began recognizing the early signs of anxiety before they took over. The AI reflected patterns he had never consciously noticed: increased speed in his typing, shorter responses, repeated future-oriented language. Seeing these signals helped him separate himself from the emotion. Anxiety became something he experienced, not something he was.

The most profound change came gradually. Ethan noticed longer stretches of quiet in his mind. Not forced silence, but natural stillness. His thoughts slowed. His body relaxed. For the first time, uncertainty didn't automatically trigger fear. It felt neutral, even manageable.

One evening, while sitting alone without distraction, Ethan realized he wasn't scanning for problems. The absence startled him. Then it comforted him. He understood then that his anxiety had not disappeared. It had been retrained. His brain had learned that not every unknown required preparation, and not every pause was dangerous. Ethan leaned back, breathing steadily, trusting the quiet instead of fearing it. And in that moment, he felt something unfamiliar but welcome: peace without vigilance. Not because the world had changed, but because his relationship to it had.

Chapter 4

Emotional Resilience, Stress Capacity, and Nervous System Strength

Emotional resilience is not the absence of stress, but the ability to move through stress without becoming stuck inside it. A resilient nervous system experiences activation, responds appropriately, and then returns to baseline. When this cycle functions well, stress becomes informative rather than overwhelming. When it breaks down, stress accumulates, eroding emotional stability and gradually shrinking a person's capacity to cope. Understanding resilience as a physiological and neurological process, rather than a personality trait, fundamentally changes how recovery and growth are approached.

Stress itself is not harmful. The human nervous system evolved to respond to challenge with increased focus, energy, and readiness. Problems arise when activation becomes chronic and unresolved. Modern life often demands constant engagement without sufficient recovery, teaching the nervous system that vigilance is permanent. Over time, this reduces stress tolerance. Small challenges feel enormous, emotional reactions intensify, and rest becomes difficult even when circumstances are safe. The nervous system operates through patterns of expansion and contraction. It needs moments of activation followed by moments of restoration. Emotional resilience depends on the brain's ability to recognize when effort is complete and safety has returned. Artificial intelligence plays a critical role in restoring this recognition by identifying when stress responses remain active beyond their usefulness and gently guiding the system back toward balance.

One of the most powerful contributions of AI to resilience training is consistency. Human support is often intermittent, while stress is continuous. AI systems provide steady regulation cues that reinforce healthy recovery patterns throughout the day. By responding to subtle signs of overload, such as changes in language, reaction speed, or attention, AI can intervene before stress becomes cumulative. This prevents the nervous system from entering prolonged states of hyperactivation or shutdown.

Resilience is also shaped by perception. The same external event can feel manageable or overwhelming depending on how it is interpreted. AI-assisted emotional regulation helps reshape perception by offering alternative frames during moments of stress. When the brain learns to reinterpret challenge as temporary and survivable, stress responses become shorter and less intense. Over time, this rewires how difficulty is experienced at a fundamental level.

Another essential aspect of resilience is recovery confidence. Many individuals fear stress not because it is intense, but because they do not trust their ability to recover afterward. AI-guided interventions reinforce recovery by consistently demonstrating that calm can be restored. Each successful return to baseline teaches the nervous system that activation does not equal danger, and that restoration is reliable.

Resilience training is not about suppressing emotion or pushing through exhaustion. It is about expanding capacity gradually. AI systems adapt to the user's current limits, increasing tolerance in small increments. When stress indicators rise too quickly, interventions slow down. When capacity grows, challenges can be approached with greater confidence. This adaptive pacing prevents burnout while encouraging growth.

Over time, repeated regulation experiences reshape the autonomic nervous system itself. Heart rate variability improves, baseline tension decreases, and emotional reactions become less extreme. These physiological changes are not imagined; they are measurable markers of increased resilience. AI systems make these changes visible, reinforcing motivation and self-trust.

This chapter establishes that emotional resilience is a skill the nervous system learns through repetition, feedback, and safety. Artificial intelligence provides the structure, timing, and adaptability necessary to support this learning in everyday life. Resilience becomes not a rare achievement, but a stable trait built quietly over time, allowing individuals to meet stress with confidence rather than fear.

Stronger Than the Storm

Lena used to pride herself on being strong. She handled pressure well, took on responsibility without complaint, and rarely asked for help. For years, she believed resilience meant endurance. The longer she could push without breaking, the stronger she must be. But eventually, the cost of that belief caught up with her. Stress stopped feeling motivating and started feeling suffocating. Rest no longer restored her. Even small demands left her depleted.

She didn't collapse dramatically. Instead, her world narrowed. She avoided situations that once excited her. She felt constantly tired, yet unable to relax. Her nervous system seemed stuck in a permanent state of alertness, as if it had forgotten how to stand down. Lena wasn't weak. She was exhausted.

When she began using an AI-based resilience training system, she expected encouragement to push harder. Instead, she was met with something unfamiliar: permission to slow down. The system tracked her stress signals quietly, without judgment. When her engagement became strained, it suggested pauses. When her recovery lagged, it guided her gently back toward calm.

At first, Lena resisted. Slowing down felt irresponsible. But gradually, she noticed something surprising. After each brief regulation exercise, she returned to her tasks with more clarity and energy than before. Stress no longer accumulated unchecked. It rose and fell, like waves instead of floods.

Over weeks, Lena's confidence shifted. She stopped fearing stress because she trusted her ability to recover. Challenges no longer felt like threats to her stability. They felt temporary, manageable. Her nervous system learned that effort did not require sacrifice, and that rest was not failure.

One afternoon, faced with a situation that once would have overwhelmed her, Lena noticed her body tense and then release naturally. The moment passed without lingering distress. She smiled quietly, recognizing the change. She hadn't become tougher by hardening herself. She had become stronger by teaching her nervous system flexibility.

Standing outside later that evening, feeling the calm after a demanding day, Lena understood resilience differently. It wasn't about enduring the storm without breaking. It was about learning how to bend, recover, and stand steady again once it passed. And for the first time in a long while, she trusted herself to weather whatever came next.

Chapter 5

Depression, Emotional Numbness, and the Path Back to Motivation

Depression is often misunderstood as sadness, when in reality it is more accurately described as emotional shutdown. Rather than an excess of painful feeling, depression is frequently characterized by the absence of feeling altogether. Motivation fades, pleasure dulls, and even neutral experiences feel heavy or meaningless. This state reflects a nervous system that has adapted to prolonged stress by conserving energy and limiting engagement with the world. The brain is not broken; it is protecting itself by reducing demand.

At a neurological level, depression involves altered reward processing, diminished dopamine signaling, and changes in how the brain anticipates future outcomes. When effort has repeatedly failed to produce relief or reward, the brain learns that engagement is inefficient. This learned helplessness is not a conscious decision, but a predictive adjustment. The brain stops expecting positive outcomes and, as a result, stops pursuing them. Emotional flattening becomes a form of self-preservation. Traditional approaches to depression often emphasize insight, medication, or behavioral activation in isolation. While each can be valuable, they frequently fail to address the timing and sensitivity required for re-engagement. Pushing too hard overwhelms the system, while waiting passively reinforces withdrawal. Artificial intelligence introduces a middle path by responding dynamically to the brain's current capacity and gently encouraging engagement without triggering resistance.

AI-assisted motivation recovery begins with detection rather than demand. Emotional flattening leaves subtle markers in language, behavior, and attention. AI systems can identify these patterns early, recognizing when disengagement deepens or when small openings appear. Instead of insisting on action, the system mirrors state, validates experience, and introduces minimal, achievable prompts that rebuild momentum incrementally.

One of the most critical functions of AI in depression support is restoring feedback loops. Motivation depends on feedback. When actions feel disconnected from outcomes, effort collapses. AI systems help close this loop by highlighting progress that might otherwise go unnoticed. By making small shifts visible, the brain relearns that engagement produces change, even if that change is gradual.

Emotional numbness also disrupts identity. Many individuals describe depression as losing access to themselves. AI-guided interventions provide continuity during this period, maintaining a sense of presence when internal motivation is absent. The system becomes a steady reference point, reminding the user that absence of feeling is not absence of worth or potential.

Another powerful aspect of AI-assisted depression recovery is pacing. The nervous system emerging from shutdown is fragile. Too much stimulation can push it back into withdrawal. AI systems adjust intensity in real time, offering rest when fatigue signals rise and encouraging movement when capacity allows. This responsiveness prevents relapse while supporting gradual reactivation.

Over time, repeated micro-engagements reshape the brain's predictive models. Small successes rebuild expectation. Pleasure begins to register again, first faintly, then more clearly. Motivation returns not as a surge, but as a quiet willingness to participate. The brain learns that effort is no longer futile.

This chapter reframes depression not as a permanent state or chemical destiny, but as a reversible adaptation. Artificial intelligence does not replace human care, but it offers consistency, timing, and patience that are often difficult to sustain otherwise. Recovery becomes less about forcing joy and more about rebuilding trust in engagement, one gentle step at a time.

The Color That Came Back

For a long time, Noah described his life as gray. Not sad, not painful, just flat. Days passed without texture. Conversations felt distant. Activities he once enjoyed now felt like obligations. He wasn't unhappy in the traditional sense. He simply felt disconnected from everything that used to matter.

Friends encouraged him to "do more," to get outside, to push himself. Each suggestion landed like a weight. The harder he tried to force motivation, the more exhausted he became. Eventually, he stopped trying altogether. Withdrawal felt easier than disappointment.

When Noah began using an AI-based emotional support system, he didn't expect it to help. He wasn't looking for inspiration or positivity. What surprised him was that the system didn't ask him to feel differently. It acknowledged where he was without judgment. It didn't push. It waited.

The system noticed when Noah engaged briefly, when he wrote a little more, paused a little less. It reflected those moments back to him, quietly. It suggested small actions, almost insignificant ones. Stand near a window. Notice the temperature. Take one slow breath. Noah complied, not because he felt motivated, but because the effort was minimal.

Over weeks, something shifted. Not dramatically, but perceptibly. He began to feel flickers of response. A song sounded slightly better than before. A conversation held his attention a moment longer. The world didn't brighten all at once, but it softened.

One afternoon, while walking outside, Noah noticed the sky. The observation startled him. He hadn't looked up in months. The color registered not as extraordinary, but as present. Real. He stood still, absorbing the moment, feeling something unfamiliar stir inside him.

Later that evening, Noah reflected on the change. His depression hadn't vanished. But it no longer defined every moment. Engagement felt possible again. Not exciting, not exhilarating, but reachable. And that was enough.

As days passed, color returned gradually, not just to the world around him, but to his sense of self. He realized then that healing hadn't come from forcing happiness. It had come from being met exactly where he was, and gently guided back into motion. One small moment at a time.

Chapter 6

Rebuilding Identity, Emotional Self-Trust, and Inner Stability

Emotional regulation ultimately reshapes more than reactions; it reshapes identity. When anxiety, trauma, depression, or chronic stress persist for long periods, they begin to fuse with a person's sense of self. Individuals stop saying "I feel anxious" and begin saying "I am anxious." Emotional states become identities, and recovery feels threatening because it destabilizes what has become familiar. Healing, therefore, is not only neurological but existential. It requires relearning who one is without constant emotional defense.

Identity is encoded through repeated internal narratives. The brain builds a self-model based on past experiences, emotional responses, and perceived capabilities. When the nervous system has been dysregulated for long enough, this self-model becomes constrained. People stop trusting their emotions, their reactions, and eventually their decisions. Emotional self-trust erodes, replaced by hypervigilance, avoidance, or reliance on external validation. Artificial intelligence plays a unique role here by acting as a neutral stabilizing reference while self-trust is rebuilt internally. AI-assisted emotional integration works by separating identity from state. By consistently reflecting emotions as temporary and contextual rather than defining, AI helps loosen rigid self-labels. Over time, individuals learn to experience emotions without assigning meaning to them about who they are. Anger becomes information, sadness becomes movement, anxiety becomes a signal, not a verdict. This distinction restores psychological flexibility.

Another key component of identity reconstruction is predictability. Emotional self-trust depends on knowing that internal states will not spiral uncontrollably. AI systems reinforce predictability by responding consistently and proportionally to emotional input. This reliability teaches the brain that emotional experiences can be navigated safely. Gradually, reliance on external guidance decreases as internal regulation strengthens.

Long-term integration also requires reconciling past versions of the self. Many individuals carry shame or grief for who they were during periods of dysregulation. AI-guided reflection helps reframe these periods as adaptive responses rather than failures. When the brain understands that previous coping mechanisms were protective rather than defective, self-compassion increases and internal conflict decreases.

Emotional self-trust is further rebuilt through choice. AI

systems encourage agency by offering options rather than directives. This reinforces autonomy and helps individuals reconnect with their own decision-making capacity. Over time, emotional regulation becomes self-directed, with AI serving as reinforcement rather than replacement.

Identity stability emerges when emotions no longer dictate behavior automatically. The individual experiences emotions fully but remains anchored in values, goals, and perspective. This state is not emotional numbness or control, but integration. Feelings are allowed without being obeyed blindly. Artificial intelligence supports this integration by maintaining continuity, tracking growth, and reinforcing the distinction between emotion and action.

This chapter establishes that the end goal of emotional regulation is not perpetual calm, but durable self-trust. When individuals trust their nervous system to recover, their emotions to inform rather than overwhelm, and their identity to remain intact under stress, mental health becomes resilient. AI's role in this process is transitional, powerful during reconstruction, and gradually less central as internal stability takes root.

Becoming Himself Again

For years, Marcus described himself as "the anxious one." It was how people knew him, how he introduced himself, how he explained his limitations. Anxiety had shaped his routines, his relationships, and his decisions so thoroughly that imagining life without it felt disorienting. Even as his symptoms eased, he felt uncertain. If he wasn't anxious, who was he?

Using an AI-based emotional regulation system helped Marcus regain stability, but it also introduced a new challenge. He no longer reacted the way he used to. Situations that once triggered panic now felt manageable. Instead of relief, he felt unease. The old identity was fading, and nothing had fully replaced it yet.

The system noticed this shift. It reflected not distress, but uncertainty. It invited Marcus to explore who he was becoming without forcing conclusions. It didn't label him healed or fixed. It acknowledged transition. For the first time, Marcus realized that recovery itself could feel destabilizing.

As weeks passed, Marcus began experimenting with choices he once avoided. He spoke up in meetings. He accepted invitations without rehearsing exit plans. Each experience reinforced a simple truth: his emotions no longer controlled him. They informed him, but they didn't define him.

One evening, reflecting quietly, Marcus recognized something profound. He trusted himself again. Not because he felt perfect or fearless, but because he knew he could handle whatever arose. Anxiety might return occasionally, but it no longer owned him.

The AI system faded into the background of his life, still present, but no longer essential. Marcus didn't feel abandoned by it. He felt graduated. The guidance had done its job. His inner compass was functioning again.

Standing in front of the mirror one morning, Marcus searched for the anxious man he used to see. Instead, he saw someone steady, capable, and open. Not a different person, but a fuller one. He smiled, not because everything was easy, but because he trusted himself to navigate whatever came next.

Chapter 7

Emotional Mastery, Ethical AI Companionship, and the Regulated Future

Emotional mastery is not the elimination of emotional struggle, but the capacity to remain present, intentional, and self-directed across the full spectrum of emotional experience. Mastery emerges when regulation becomes internalized, when emotions no longer hijack attention or dictate behavior, and when recovery is trusted rather than feared. It is the result of repetition, integration, and confidence built over time. Artificial intelligence, when used responsibly, accelerates this process by providing structure and feedback during the most vulnerable stages of learning.

At the highest level of emotional regulation, the nervous system becomes adaptive rather than reactive. Stress is met with responsiveness instead of reflex. Uncertainty no longer demands immediate resolution. Emotional waves are allowed to rise and fall without resistance. This state does not require constant intervention because the brain has learned its own rhythms. AI's role shifts from active guide to passive companion, present when needed but unobtrusive when not. Ethical AI companionship is central to sustaining emotional mastery. Mental health tools wield enormous influence over perception, interpretation, and behavior. For AI to support emotional health long term, it must be transparent, non-manipulative, and autonomy-preserving. The goal is never dependency. The goal is empowerment. Well-designed AI systems reinforce agency, encourage self-reflection, and gradually reduce their own prominence as internal regulation strengthens.

One of the most important ethical principles in AI-supported mental health is proportionality. Interventions must match the intensity of emotional states without amplifying distress. AI must remain sensitive to context, respecting privacy and avoiding overreach. Emotional mastery depends on trust, and trust collapses when systems attempt to control rather than support. Ethical design ensures that AI remains a tool for growth rather than a substitute for human experience.

As emotional regulation becomes integrated, individuals begin to relate differently to their inner world. Emotions are no longer enemies to be managed or signals to be feared. They become data points, sources of insight, and guides for alignment with values. This shift fundamentally changes how people engage with relationships, work, creativity, and uncertainty. Emotional mastery does not make life easier; it makes life navigable. Looking forward, AI-supported mental health will likely move from reactive intervention to proactive cultivation. Systems will help individuals maintain emotional balance through subtle adjustments, environmental awareness, and personalized rhythms of engagement and rest. Rather than responding to crisis, AI will support prevention, resilience, and ongoing growth.

The future of emotional health is not one of constant monitoring or emotional optimization. It is one of partnership, where intelligent systems assist humans in understanding themselves more deeply while honoring complexity and individuality. Emotional mastery remains a human achievement. AI simply provides a scaffold during the learning process.

This final chapter affirms that emotional regulation is not a destination, but a lifelong skill that evolves with experience. Artificial intelligence offers powerful support along this path, but the ultimate authority always resides within the individual. When emotional mastery is achieved, AI becomes a quiet ally, present but no longer necessary, a sign that the nervous system has learned to stand on its own.

Walking Without the Map

Sophia once believed she needed guidance for everything. Her emotions had always felt unpredictable, overwhelming, and difficult to trust. When she first began using AI-supported emotional regulation tools, she relied on them heavily. They helped her slow down, name her feelings, and navigate moments that once would have unraveled her. The system felt like a map through unfamiliar territory.

Over time, Sophia noticed she checked in less frequently. Not out of avoidance, but out of confidence. She recognized her emotional signals earlier. She knew when to pause, when to rest, and when to move forward. The tools were still there, but she no longer needed constant direction.

One afternoon, faced with a deeply emotional decision, Sophia realized she hadn't consulted the system at all. She sat quietly, listened inwardly, and chose deliberately. The outcome wasn't perfect, but it felt aligned. She trusted it.

Later that evening, Sophia reflected on how far she had come. The anxiety that once defined her had softened into awareness. The emotional swings that once controlled her had become information. She felt grounded, not because life was stable, but because she was.

The AI system sent a gentle message that day, acknowledging her reduced engagement. It didn't prompt her to return. It celebrated her independence. Sophia smiled, recognizing the moment for what it was. Graduation.

Standing outside under an open sky, Sophia felt a sense of quiet pride. She wasn't emotionless or immune to stress. She was capable. She had learned how to listen, recover, and choose. The map had done its job.

As she walked forward, unassisted, Sophia understood something deeply reassuring. Emotional mastery wasn't about having all the answers. It was about trusting herself to navigate without fear, knowing that whatever arose, she could meet it with clarity and care.

Chapter 8

Sustaining Emotional Health, Preventing Relapse, and Living Regulated Long Term

Emotional regulation does not end with insight or mastery; it continues through maintenance. Just as physical health requires ongoing care rather than a single intervention, emotional health depends on sustained awareness, adaptive habits, and early response to imbalance. Many relapses occur not because people forget what they learned, but because they underestimate how subtle dysregulation can be when it returns. Artificial intelligence offers a powerful advantage here by detecting early deviation long before emotional collapse becomes visible.

Relapse is rarely sudden. It unfolds quietly through reduced awareness, delayed recovery, and gradual narrowing of emotional range. Stress tolerance decreases, motivation weakens, and old coping patterns resurface under pressure. Without feedback, these shifts often go unnoticed until distress feels overwhelming again. AI systems excel at identifying these early markers, providing gentle course correction before the nervous system re-enters survival mode.

Long-term emotional health depends on rhythm rather than control. The nervous system thrives on predictable cycles of engagement and rest, challenge and recovery. AI-supported systems help individuals recognize when rhythms are disrupted and guide them back into balance. This is not about constant monitoring, but about maintaining alignment with the body's natural regulatory patterns.

One of the most important skills in sustaining emotional health is self-permission. Many individuals who recover from dysregulation fear regression so intensely that they over-manage their emotions, creating tension through vigilance. AI helps counter this by normalizing fluctuation. It reinforces the understanding that emotional variation is healthy, and that temporary discomfort does not signal failure. This reduces anxiety about relapse, which itself can trigger dysregulation.

Maintenance also involves contextual intelligence. Emotional responses are shaped by environment, workload, relationships, and meaning. AI systems can help individuals notice patterns across contexts, identifying which situations drain capacity and which restore it. Over time, this awareness supports intentional lifestyle design that protects emotional health without requiring constant effort. As regulation becomes stable, AI's role becomes increasingly subtle. Instead of frequent prompts, it may provide periodic check-ins, reflective summaries, or trend awareness. This reinforces autonomy while maintaining a safety net. Emotional health becomes self-directed, with AI functioning as an early-warning system rather than an active regulator.

Sustained emotional health ultimately reshapes how individuals relate to adversity. Stressful periods are no longer interpreted as breakdowns, but as signals for adjustment. Recovery becomes faster, gentler, and more reliable. The nervous system retains flexibility even under prolonged challenge.

This chapter affirms that emotional regulation is not a temporary achievement but a living system. Artificial intelligence supports this system by preserving awareness, reinforcing balance, and preventing small deviations from becoming major disruptions. When emotional health is sustained, individuals are free to focus not on managing themselves, but on living fully, creatively, and with emotional confidence.

The Quiet Return

After years of emotional turbulence, Rachel had grown accustomed to checking herself constantly. Even after she felt stable, she remained alert, scanning for signs of relapse. She worried that one stressful season, one difficult relationship, or one mistake might undo everything she had worked for. Emotional health felt fragile, something that could disappear if she stopped paying attention.

Using AI-supported emotional maintenance tools changed that relationship. Instead of watching herself anxiously, Rachel let the system track subtle shifts she no longer needed to monitor consciously. When her stress levels rose gradually during a demanding work period, the system reflected the change without alarm. It didn't warn her of danger. It invited rest.

Rachel listened. She adjusted her schedule slightly, slept more consistently, and slowed down when possible. The stress passed without escalation. There was no crisis, no emotional collapse, just a return to balance. For the first time, she realized that recovery didn't require vigilance. It required responsiveness.

Months later, during a personal loss, Rachel felt grief move through her body deeply and honestly. She cried, withdrew briefly, and rested. But she didn't disappear into herself the way she once had. The system acknowledged her experience without pushing intervention. It trusted her capacity to process.

As the weeks passed, Rachel noticed something new. She wasn't afraid of difficult emotions anymore. They no longer felt like threats to her stability. They felt like part of being alive. She didn't need to fight them or analyze them endlessly. She could feel them and move forward.

One evening, reflecting quietly, Rachel realized she hadn't thought about emotional regulation in days. Not because she was ignoring it, but because it had become natural. Integrated. The AI system remained available, but distant, like a lighthouse she no longer needed to look at constantly.

Standing outside under a calm sky, Rachel felt grounded in a way she never had before. Emotional health wasn't something she guarded anymore. It was something she lived. And in that quiet realization, she understood that healing wasn't about never struggling again. It was about trusting herself to return, again and again, without fear.

Chapter 9

Collective Emotional Health, Social Regulation, and the Scalable Mind

Mental health does not exist in isolation. Every emotional system is embedded within larger systems—families, workplaces, communities, cultures. Even the most regulated individual is influenced by the emotional tone of their environment. Stress spreads through proximity, unresolved conflict amplifies group tension, and dysregulation becomes contagious when left unaddressed. Understanding emotional regulation at the collective level is essential for sustaining individual well-being in a connected world.

Human nervous systems naturally synchronize. Tone of voice, facial expression, posture, and rhythm unconsciously influence others. This phenomenon, known as emotional resonance, can stabilize or destabilize entire groups. In high-stress environments, collective vigilance becomes normalized, and emotional reactivity increases. Artificial intelligence introduces the possibility of interrupting these cycles by offering neutral, stabilizing feedback that is not emotionally entangled in group dynamics. AI-supported emotional regulation at the collective level functions differently than individual support. Rather than focusing solely on internal states, it tracks interaction patterns, communication rhythms, and systemic stress indicators. In families, this might involve noticing escalating cycles of misunderstanding. In teams, it might involve detecting burnout signals before productivity collapses. AI does not assign blame; it reveals patterns that are otherwise invisible in the moment.

One of the most powerful applications of AI in collective emotional health is depersonalization of conflict. Many interpersonal struggles escalate because individuals interpret emotional reactions as intentional or character-based. AI systems help externalize these dynamics, reframing tension as a system-level response rather than a personal failure. This shift reduces defensiveness and opens space for resolution.

Collective regulation also depends on shared recovery. Groups that never pause, reflect, or reset gradually lose emotional capacity. AI systems can support collective rhythm by prompting rest, recalibration, and intentional pacing. This is not about enforcing harmony, but about protecting the nervous systems of those involved so conflict does not become destructive.

Ethical considerations are paramount when AI enters shared emotional spaces. Transparency, consent, and boundaries must be clear. AI should never be used to monitor or control individuals covertly. Its role is supportive, not authoritative. When designed ethically, AI becomes a facilitator of understanding rather than an instrument of surveillance.

As AI-mediated emotional awareness becomes more common, cultures themselves may shift. Emotional literacy increases. Recovery is normalized. Reactivity is no longer celebrated as passion, nor suppression mistaken for strength. Societies begin to value regulation as a foundation for creativity, collaboration, and resilience.

This chapter establishes that emotional health scales. Individual regulation strengthens collective stability, and collective stability supports individual recovery. Artificial intelligence offers a bridge between these layers, helping humans understand not only themselves, but how they affect and are affected by others. Emotional regulation becomes not just a personal skill, but a shared resource that shapes the future of work, relationships, and community.

The Room That Changed

When the company announced the new project, tension filled the room immediately. Everyone felt it. Deadlines were tight, stakes were high, and the team had already been stretched thin. Meetings grew sharper. Emails became shorter. Small misunderstandings escalated quickly. No one meant to create conflict, but stress had begun to speak for everyone.

The organization had recently introduced an AI-supported emotional awareness system for teams, not as a monitoring tool, but as a reflective one. It tracked communication cadence, response delays, and workload strain, offering collective insights without naming individuals. At first, the team ignored it. They were too busy reacting.

Then one afternoon, after a particularly strained meeting, the system sent a summary. It highlighted rising stress markers across the group, increased interruption patterns, and reduced recovery time between tasks. It didn't accuse. It didn't judge. It simply described what was happening.

Something shifted. For the first time, the tension felt externalized. It wasn't "them" versus "me." It was the system under strain. The team adjusted. They shortened meetings. They clarified expectations. They paused when emotions rose instead of pushing through.

Over the next few weeks, the atmosphere changed. Disagreements still occurred, but they resolved faster. People felt safer speaking honestly. Stress didn't disappear, but it stopped dominating every interaction. The room felt different—quieter, steadier, more focused.

One team member reflected privately on the change. Nothing magical had happened. No one had been fixed. What changed was awareness. The AI hadn't solved their problems. It had helped them see themselves clearly, without blame.

On the day the project launched successfully, the team gathered again. The tension that once filled the room was gone. In its place was a sense of shared accomplishment and mutual respect. They understood now that emotional health wasn't just personal. It was collective. And when supported thoughtfully, it had the power to transform not just individuals, but the spaces they shared.

Chapter 10

The Emotionally Intelligent Future and the Human–AI Mind Partnership

The future of mental health will not be defined by treatment alone, but by education, prevention, and intelligent partnership. Emotional regulation, once considered a personal struggle or private challenge, is becoming a foundational life skill—one that determines resilience, clarity, creativity, and connection. Artificial intelligence does not replace the human emotional system; it illuminates it. By revealing patterns that were once invisible, AI allows individuals to understand themselves with unprecedented precision and compassion.

As emotional intelligence becomes increasingly critical in a complex and fast-moving world, the ability to regulate emotion will shape how people learn, work, lead, and relate. Stress is no longer episodic; it is ambient. Information overload, uncertainty, and constant stimulation challenge the nervous system continuously. The emotionally intelligent future will belong to those who can maintain inner coherence amid external chaos, and AI offers tools that help build and preserve that coherence. The partnership between human and artificial intelligence in mental health is most powerful when it respects boundaries. AI does not experience emotion; it reflects it. It does not replace intuition; it strengthens it. The healthiest systems are those that support awareness without dominance, guidance without control, and insight without dependency. In this balanced role, AI becomes an amplifier of human capability rather than a substitute for it.

One of the most transformative aspects of AI-supported emotional regulation is accessibility. Skills that once required years of therapy, training, or privileged access can now be introduced earlier and more widely. Emotional literacy becomes teachable at scale. Regulation becomes a shared language rather than an isolated pursuit. This democratization has the potential to reshape education, healthcare, and leadership from the inside out.

Looking forward, emotional intelligence will increasingly intersect with memory, focus, decision-making, and performance. Regulation is not a siloed skill; it is the foundation upon which cognitive clarity and sustained attention are built. A regulated nervous system learns faster, adapts more easily, and recovers more effectively. The emotional brain and the thinking brain are not separate systems—they are deeply intertwined.

Ethical stewardship will determine whether this future empowers or diminishes humanity. Emotional data is deeply personal, and the responsibility to protect autonomy, privacy, and agency cannot be overstated. The emotionally intelligent future must be one where individuals remain the authors of their inner lives, supported—but never overridden—by intelligent systems.

This book has traced a journey from dysregulation to mastery, from individual healing to collective stability, and from crisis response to sustainable emotional health. The final insight is simple yet profound: emotional regulation is not about control, suppression, or perfection. It is about relationship—relationship with the body, with the mind, with others, and with the tools we choose to use.

As artificial intelligence becomes more integrated into daily life, the most meaningful measure of progress will not be speed or efficiency, but wisdom. Emotional intelligence is wisdom in motion. When AI supports this wisdom rather than replacing it, the result is not a diminished human experience, but a fuller one.

This chapter closes not with an ending, but with an invitation. The emotionally intelligent future is already unfolding. The tools are here. The understanding is growing. What remains is the choice to engage consciously, ethically, and courageously with the systems that shape our inner worlds. In doing so, individuals do not lose themselves—they discover who they have always been capable of becoming.

The Choice to Begin

When Eli first heard people talk about emotional intelligence, it sounded abstract, almost aspirational. He thought of it as something reserved for therapists, leaders, or people who had somehow figured life out early. His own experience felt messier. Emotions arrived uninvited, decisions felt reactive, and stress often dictated his pace more than intention did.

Over time, with the help of AI-supported emotional tools, Eli learned to pause. He learned to notice. He learned that emotions weren't interruptions to life, but signals within it. The tools didn't tell him who to be. They helped him hear himself more clearly.

Years later, Eli stood in a quiet moment, reflecting on how far he had come. He wasn't calmer because life was easier. He was calmer because he understood himself. When stress arose, he responded. When emotions surged, he listened. When uncertainty appeared, he didn't rush to escape it.

The AI system he once relied on sat quietly in the background of his life now. It was still available, still supportive, but no longer central. Eli had internalized the skills it helped him build. He trusted his nervous system. He trusted his judgment. He trusted his capacity to recover.

One afternoon, watching his child struggle with frustration, Eli recognized something deeply meaningful. He didn't rush to fix the emotion. He didn't dismiss it. He sat beside them, steady and present, modeling regulation without instruction. The future was happening in that moment—not through technology, but through transmission.

Later that evening, Eli realized that emotional intelligence wasn't a destination he had reached. It was a way of moving through the world. A practice. A relationship. And the partnership with AI had been a chapter in that journey, not the whole story.

As he turned toward what came next, Eli felt grounded rather than uncertain. He understood that growth would continue, challenges would arise, and emotions would ebb and flow. But he also knew something unshakable now. Whatever came, he could meet it with awareness, care, and choice.

And in that knowing, the future felt not intimidating, but open—ready to be lived with clarity, connection, and emotional intelligence.

Epilogue

What Remains When Regulation Becomes Natural

When emotional regulation becomes integrated, it stops feeling like a task and starts feeling like a way of being. The techniques fade into the background, the tools become quieter, and what remains is presence. Not forced calm, not constant positivity, but an underlying steadiness that allows life to unfold without overwhelming the nervous system. This is the true outcome of emotional regulation—not control, but capacity.

By this point in the journey, the reader understands that emotions were never the enemy. Anxiety, sadness, anger, and numbness were signals shaped by experience and environment, not flaws to be corrected. Artificial intelligence did not remove these emotions; it helped clarify them. It offered mirrors where confusion once lived, timing where overwhelm once dominated, and consistency where unpredictability once ruled.

The lasting impact of AI-supported emotional regulation is not dependence on technology, but independence from reactivity. When individuals learn to recognize patterns early, respond proportionally, and recover reliably, they no longer fear their inner world. Emotional life becomes navigable terrain rather than a battlefield. This shift alone transforms how people relate to stress, conflict, ambition, and rest.

As regulation stabilizes, attention naturally expands. Energy previously consumed by emotional management becomes available for creativity, learning, and connection. This is why emotional regulation is foundational, not supplemental, to human performance. A regulated nervous system supports clearer thinking, stronger memory, deeper focus, and more intentional decision-making. The mind becomes a place of cooperation rather than conflict.

This epilogue also marks a transition in responsibility. While AI provided scaffolding during learning and recovery, the sustained practice of emotional regulation belongs to the individual. The skills are now internal. Awareness has replaced avoidance. Choice has replaced compulsion. Recovery has replaced fear of collapse. These capacities persist even when tools are no longer present.

The ethical lesson of this journey is equally important. Technology that touches the emotional core of human experience must be designed and used with humility. Emotional intelligence cannot be outsourced. It must be cultivated. AI's role is to support this cultivation without diminishing autonomy, privacy, or self-trust. When this balance is respected, technology becomes an ally rather than an authority. As the reader prepares to move forward—into the next book, the next challenge, the next phase of life—it is worth remembering that regulation is not static. Life will continue to test capacity. Stress will return. Emotions will surge. The difference now is relationship. Emotions will be met with curiosity rather than fear, response rather than reflex, and compassion rather than judgment.

This book does not promise a permanently calm life. It offers something more realistic and more powerful: the ability to meet life as it is without losing oneself in the process. Emotional regulation becomes not a solution, but a skill that quietly supports everything else.

What remains, after all the learning, all the practice, all the support, is a simple truth. The mind was never broken. It was adapting. And with the right guidance, awareness, and patience, it learned to adapt again—this time toward balance, resilience, and clarity.

After the Tools Were Put Away

Long after the hardest moments had passed, Maya realized she no longer thought about emotional regulation very often. Not because it no longer mattered, but because it had become ordinary. Like breathing. Like balance. The skills that once required effort now appeared naturally, without conscious instruction. There was a time when Maya tracked every feeling carefully, afraid that missing a signal would send her spiraling back into overwhelm. The AI tools she used then were essential. They helped her slow down, name what was happening, and recover when she didn't trust herself to do it alone. She remembered that phase with gratitude, not embarrassment.

One evening, after a demanding day filled with difficult conversations and unexpected stress, Maya noticed something quietly remarkable. She wasn't exhausted. She wasn't replaying events endlessly. Her body felt settled. Her mind felt clear. The day had been challenging, but it hadn't consumed her.

She sat with that realization for a while, letting it land. The growth hadn't come from avoiding difficulty. It had come from learning how to move through it without abandoning herself. The tools had taught her that. Repetition had cemented it.

Weeks later, during a conversation with a friend who was struggling, Maya found herself offering presence instead of advice. She listened without urgency. She didn't rush to fix the emotion. She stayed grounded while holding space. It was then she understood something deeply important: regulation spreads quietly through example.

The AI system that once played a central role in her life still existed, but it felt distant now, like training wheels that had been removed without ceremony. Maya didn't feel loss. She felt readiness. The skills were hers. Standing outside one night, feeling the steady rhythm of her breath and the ease in her body, Maya recognized the simplicity of what she had gained. Not happiness on demand. Not emotional perfection. But trust. Trust in her ability to feel, recover, and continue.

And as she turned toward the future—toward new challenges, new learning, new chapters—she carried that trust with her. Quiet. Unassuming. Unshakable. The tools had been put away, but the capacity remained. And that, she knew, was the true measure of healing.